CARDIO SUCKS!

THE SIMPLE SCIENCE OF BURNING FAT FAST AND GETTING IN SHAPE

Michael Matthews

oculus

Cover Designed by: Damon Freeman

Typesetting by Kiersten Lief

Published by: Oculus Publishers, Inc.

www.oculuspublishers.com

Visit the author's website:

www.muscleforlife.com

ABOUT THE AUTHOR

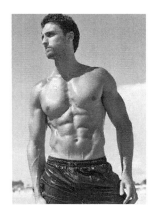

Hi,

I'm Mike and I've been training for nearly a decade now.

I believe that every person can achieve the body of his or her dreams, and I work hard to give everyone that chance by providing workable, proven advice grounded in science, not a desire to sell phony magazines, workout products, or supplements.

Through my work, I've helped thousands of people achieve their health and fitness goals, and I share everything I know in my books.

So if you're looking to get in shape and look great, then I think I can help you. I hope you enjoy my books and I'd love to hear from you at my site, www.muscleforlife.com.

Sincerely,
Mike

ALSO BY MICHAEL MATTHEWS

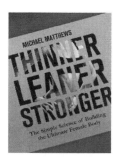

Thinner Leaner Stronger: The Simple Science of Building the Ultimate Female Body

If you want to be toned, lean, and strong as quickly as possible without crash dieting, "good genetics," or wasting ridiculous amounts of time in the gym and money on supplements...*regardless of your age...* then you want to read this book.

Visit www.muscleforlife.com to get this book!

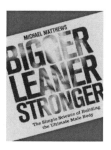

Bigger Leaner Stronger: The Simple Science of Building the Ultimate Male Body

If you want to be muscular, lean, and strong as quickly as possible, without steroids, "good genetics," or wasting ridiculous amounts of time in the gym, and money on supplements...then you want to read this book.

Visit www.muscleforlife.com to get this book!

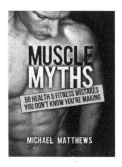

Muscle Myths: 50 Health & Fitness Mistakes You Don't Know You're Making

If you've ever felt lost in the sea of contradictory training and diet advice out there and you just want to know once and for all what works and what doesn't—what's scientifically true and what's false—when it comes to building muscle and getting ripped, then you need to read this book.

Visit www.muscleforlife.com to get this book!

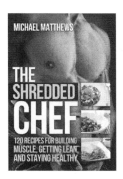

The Shredded Chef: 120 Recipes for Building Muscle, Getting Lean, and Staying Healthy

If you want to know how to forever escape the dreadful experience of "dieting" and learn how to cook nutritious, delicious meals that make building muscle and burning fat easy and enjoyable, then you need to read this book.

Visit www.muscleforlife.com to get this book!

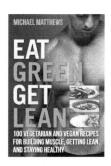

Eat Green Get Lean: 100 Vegetarian and Vegan Recipes for Building Muscle, Getting Lean, and Staying Healthy

If you want to know how to build muscle and burn fat by eating delicious vegetarian and vegan meals that are easy to cook and easy on your wallet, then you want to read this book.

Visit www.muscleforlife.com to learn more about this book!

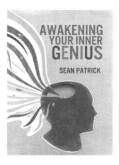

Awakening Your Inner Genius

If you'd like to know what some of history's greatest thinkers and achievers can teach you about awakening your inner genius, and how to find, follow, and fulfill your journey to greatness, then you want to read this book today.

(I'm using a pen name for this book, as well as for a few other projects not related to health and fitness, but I thought you might enjoy it so I'm including it here.)

Visit www.yourinnergenius.com to learn more about this book!

CONTENTS

It's time for serious fat loss soldier! This circuit training routine is as tough as they come!

If you like to hike, you'll love this method of exercise. Serious calorie burning!

If you're looking to lose fat and tone up your stomach, this is the routine for you.

If you want to learn the truth about 12 myths and mistakes that ruin people's efforts to get fit, get this free report.

You're awesome for reading my book, and I have a small favor to ask...

YOU DON'T NEED LONG, GRUELING WORKOUTS TO GET INTO GREAT SHAPE

YOU'RE FAST ASLEEP IN YOUR bed. You're warm, relaxed, and enjoying a dream that you hope never ends.

A clanging sound jolts you from your slumber. You look out of the window and the sun is peeking over the horizon.

Why the heck is your alarm set so early? Because you have to do your cardio. Ugh!

Or maybe you experience the other version of this dreadful feeling. The one where it's the evening and you're at home on the couch, winding down after a long day. Your belly is full of food and maybe some wine, and you finally feel like you're catching a breather. And then you're supposed to rev your energy back up and go for a jog.

Well, let's face it. For most of us, cardio sucks. One of the biggest reasons people fail with exercise is that they have too much trouble fitting it into their schedule. But we know that regular cardiovascular exercise is a big factor in losing weight, so what are we to do? How can we get better motivated and see better results?

That's what this book is all about. If you know what you're doing, you can not only spend less time exercising and burn more fat, but you can also actually have some *fun* in the process. (And you don't have to step foot in a gym.)

Cardio isn't complicated, and these methods don't need a ton of information to fill up the pages. But you need to know some important principles of exercise and fat loss to get the most out of your training from the least amount of time and effort. And, as you'll see, there are quite a few fun ways to achieve this.

Chances are you'll find some of these methods tougher than those you're used to. But keep in mind that they'll also take less time, and you'll get more out of them in the end. So, I think you'll find them worth the extra effort.

I'm also going to share with you some common misconceptions people have about losing weight and the simple principles of burning fat. I think this information will help you achieve your fitness goals.

So let's get started.

1

THE FOUR BIGGEST FAT LOSS MYTHS AND MISTAKES

WITH OBESITY RATES OVER 33 percent here in America (and steadily rising), it would appear that getting into great shape must require a level of knowledge, discipline, and sacrifice beyond that of which most humans are capable.

Well, this simply isn't true. The knowledge is easy enough to understand (in fact, you're learning everything you need to know in this book). Sure, it requires discipline and some "sacrifice" in that no, you can't eat three pizzas a week and have a six pack. But here's the kicker: When you're training and dieting correctly, you will *enjoy* the lifestyle; you will look forward to your exercise; you won't mind watching what you eat; and you won't feel compelled to eat junk food or desserts (even though you will be able to have them).

Simply put: You will look and feel better than you ever have before—and this will continue to improve every month—and you will find it infinitely more pleasurable and valuable than being lazy and addicted to ice cream and potato chips. When you can get into this "zone," you can do whatever you want with your body—the results are inevitable; it's just a matter of time.

But most people never find this sweet spot. Why? Well, the most practical answer to that question is twofold: First, they don't have a strong enough desire to get there (they don't have their "inner game" sorted out), and second, they lack the know-how required to make it happen, which leads to poor results, which kills discipline and makes sacrifices no longer worthwhile.

In this chapter, I want to address the five most common myths and mistakes of burning fat. Like those of building muscle, these fallacies and errors have snuck into our heads via magazines, advertising, trainers, friends, etc. Let's dispel them once and for all so that they can't block your path to having the lean body that you desire.

MYTH & MISTAKE #1:
COUNTING CALORIES IS UNNECESSARY

I don't know how many people I've consulted who wanted to lose weight but didn't want to have to count calories. This statement is about as logical as saying that they want to drive across the country but don't want to have to pay attention to their gas tank.

Now, I won't be too hard on them because they didn't even know what a calorie was, and they just didn't want to be bothered with having to count something. Well, whether you want to call it "counting" calories or whatever else, in order to lose weight, you have to regulate food intake.

In order to lose fat, you must keep your body burning more energy than you're feeding it, and the energy potential of food is measured in calories. Eat too many calories—give your body more potential energy than it needs—and it has no incentive to burn fat.

What people are actually objecting to with counting calories is trying to figure out what to eat while on the run every day or what to buy when rushing through the grocery store. When they have a 30-minute window for lunch and run to the nearest restaurant, they don't want to have to analyze the menu to figure out calories. They just order something that sounds healthy and hope for the best. But, little do they know that their quick, "healthy" meal has hundreds of more calories than they should've eaten. Repeat that for dinner, and a day of weight loss progress is totally lost.

Well, that's the problem—not "having to counting calories." They are making it unnecessarily hard by failing to plan and prepare meals. It might seem easier to just heat up a big plate of leftovers or grab Chipotle for lunch and carry on with your day, but that convenience comes with a price: little or no weight loss.

MYTH & MISTAKE #2:
DO CARDIO = LOSE WEIGHT

Every day I see overweight people grinding away on the cardio machines. And, week after week goes by with them looking fatter than ever.

They are under the false impression that idly going through the motions on an elliptical machine or stationary bike will somehow flip a magical fat loss switch in the body. Well, that's not how it works.

You already know how to lose fat (make your body burn more energy than it gets from food), and cardio can *enhance* fat loss in two ways: 1) by burning calories and 2) by speeding up your metabolic rate.

To clarify point #2, your body burns a certain number of calories regardless of any physical activity, and this is called your *basal metabolic rate*. Your total caloric expenditure for a day would be your BMR plus the energy expended during any physical activities.

When your metabolism is said to "speed up" or "slow down," what this means is that your basal metabolic rate has gone up or down. That is, your body is burning more calories while at rest (allowing you to eat more calories without putting on fat) or burning less (making it easier to eat too much and gain fat).

But here's the thing with cardio: If you don't eat correctly, that nightly run or bike ride won't necessarily save you.

Let's say you're trying to lose weight and are unwittingly eating six hundred calories more than your body burns during the day. You go jogging for thirty minutes at night, which burns about three hundred calories. That leaves you with a daily excess of three hundred calories, and the small jump in your metabolic rate from the cardio won't be enough to burn that up *plus* burn fat stores.

You could continue like this for years and never get lean. As a matter of fact, you'll probably slowly put on weight instead.

MYTH & MISTAKE #3:
CHASING THE FADS

The Atkins Diet. The South Beach Diet. The Paleo Diet. The HCG Diet (this one really makes me cringe). The Hollywood Diet. The Body Type Diet. It seems like a new one pops up every month or two. I can't keep up these days.

While not all "latest and greatest" diets are bad (Paleo is quite healthy, actually), the sheer abundance of fad diets being touted by ripped actors is making people pretty confused as to what the "right way" to lose weight is (and understandably so).

The result is that many people jump from diet to diet, failing to get the results they desire. And, they buy into some pretty stupid stuff simply because they don't understand the physiology of metabolism and fat loss.

The rules are the rules, and no fancy names or snake oil supplements will help you get around them.

In this book, you're going to learn how simple getting ripped really is. Once you understand the basic principles of why the body stores fat and how to coax it into shedding it, you'll see how asinine many of the fad diets taking gyms by storm really are.

MYTH & MISTAKE #4:
DOING LOW WEIGHT AND HIGH REPS GETS YOU TONED

This myth goes like this: If you want that lean, toned look, you want to do a BUNCH of reps with low weight. This is just plain wrong.

To be honest, I can't think of a reason why anyone would want to do a routine based on low weight and high reps. While there's a never-ending debate as to what rep ranges are best for hypertrophy (muscle growth), many studies agree that doing more than fifteen reps causes little–to-no improvements in muscle strength or size due to insufficient overload.

Being shredded is a matter of having low body fat. Nothing else. Building muscle mass is a matter of overloading the muscles and letting them repair. Nothing more.

Light weights don't overload the muscles no matter how many reps you do (remember that *fatigue* doesn't trigger growth). No overload = no growth.

Heavy weights, however, do overload the muscles and force them to adapt. Optimum overload and proper nutrition and rest = fast, noticeable growth.

So, even if you don't want to gain too much muscle mass—let's say fifteen pounds—the fastest route to that goal is *heavy weight*. Once you're there, you can simply maintain what you have (more on that later).

MYTH & MISTAKE #5:
SPOT REDUCTION

How many guys have you seen doing crunches "to get a six pack"? How many girls try to target their butts and thighs to "burn away the fat"?

Well, that's not how it works. You can't reduce fat in any particular area of your body by targeting it with exercises. You can reduce fat by proper dieting, and your body will decide how it comes off (which areas will become lean first and which will be stubborn). Our bodies are all genetically programmed differently, and there's nothing we can do to change that. We all have our "fat spots" that annoy us to no end, and that's just genetics for you. Some guys I know store every last pound in their hips while others are fortunate to have their fat accumulate more in their chest, shoulders, and arms more so than their waistline.

Rest assured, however, that you *can* lose as much fat all over your body as you want, and you *can* get as ripped as you want; you'll just have to be patient and let your body lean out in the way it's programmed to.

THE BOTTOM LINE

Many people approach fat loss in the completely wrong way and, thus, fail to achieve their weight goals. The laws of fat loss are actually very simple, however, and also incredibly effective. Carry on to learn the laws and how to put them to work for you.

2

THE REAL SCIENCE OF HEALTHY FAT LOSS

BEFORE GETTING INTO THE LAWS of fat loss, I want to share some insight into how your body views fat versus muscle. Your body views fat as an asset and muscle as a liability. Why?

Because evolution has taught the body that having fat means being able to survive the times when food is scarce. Many thousands of years ago, when our ancestors were roaming the wilderness, they sometimes journeyed for days without food, and their bodies lived off fat stores. Starving, they would finally kill an animal and feast, and their bodies knew to prepare for the next bout of starvation by storing fat. Having fat was literally a matter of life and death.

This genetic programming is still in us, ready to be used. If you starve your body, it will burn fat to stay alive, but it will also slow down its metabolic rate to conserve energy, becoming fully prepared to store fat once you start feeding it higher quantities of food again.

Muscle, on the other hand, is viewed as a liability because it costs energy to maintain. While there is much debate as to the exact numbers in terms of calories, a pound of muscle on your body burns more energy than carrying a pound of fat. Thus, your body doesn't want to carry more muscle than it has to because it knows that it has to keep it properly fed, and this requires calories that it may or may not get.

So, what does this mean for fat loss? Well, it means that you have to show your body that it has no reason to store excess fat and, in a sense, coax it to the level that you desire. Same goes for building muscle. If you don't provide your body with the perfect building conditions (proper training, proper nutrition, and proper rest), it will be inclined to simply not grow its muscles.

All right, let's dive into to the fundamental laws of fat loss.

THE FIRST LAW OF FAT LOSS: EAT LESS THAN YOU EXPEND = LOSE WEIGHT

Fat loss is just a science of numbers, much like gaining muscle. No matter what anyone tells you, getting ripped boils down to nothing more than manipulating a simple mathematical formula: energy consumed versus energy expended. As you would expect, this has been determined beyond the shadow of a doubt by many studies, including the definitive study conducted by the University of Lausanne.

When you give your body more calories (potential energy) than it burns off, it stores fat (unless your metabolism is very fast, in which case you may not store fat but won't lose it either). When you give your body less calories than it burns throughout the day, it must make up for that deficit by burning its own energy stores (fat), leading to the ultimate goal, fat loss. It doesn't even matter what you eat—if your calories are right, you'll lose weight. Don't believe me?

Professor Mark Haub, from Kansas State University, conducted a weight loss study on himself in 2010. He started the study at 211 pounds and 33.4% body fat (overweight). He calculated that he would need to eat about 1,800 calories per day to lose weight without starving himself. He followed this protocol for two months and lost 27 pounds, but here's the kicker: while he did have one protein shake and a couple servings of vegetables each day, two-thirds of his daily caories came from Twinkies, Little Debbies, Doritos, sugary cereals, and Oreos—a "convenience store diet," as he called it. And he not only lost the weight, but his "bad" cholesterol, or LDL, dropped 20 percent and his "good" cholesterol, or HDL, increased 20 percent.

Now, Haub doesn't recommend this diet, of course, but he was doing it to prove a point. When it comes to fat loss, calories are king.

Healthy fat loss isn't as simple as drastically cutting calories, however. If you eat too little, your body will go into "starvation mode" and sure, it will lose fat, but you will also lose muscle. Plus, worst of all, your metabolic rate will slow down, and once you start eating more, you'll quickly gain the fat back (and sometimes even more than you lost). This is what leads to yo-yo dieting.

So yes, you will need to watch your calories. Yes, you will get used to feeling a little hungry (at least for the first week or two of cutting). Yes, you will have to stay disciplined and skip the daily desserts. But, if you do it right, you can get absolutely *shredded* without losing muscle…or even while gaining muscle (yes, this can be done—more on that later).

THE SECOND LAW OF FAT LOSS:
EAT SMALL, FREQUENT MEALS

Most people have heard this advice before, but they don't understand why it helps.

The most common reason given for increasing meal frequency is that it increases metabolism. It makes logical sense—by putting food in our bodies every few hours, it has to constantly work to break it down, which should speed up our metabolism, right?

Well, the jury is still out on this one. Studies contradict each other left and right. Some have found that several smaller meals per day increased metabolic rates in subjects, while others found that it didn't.

What has been conclusively proven, however, is that people who consume smaller, more frequent meals each day have more success losing weight than those who eat larger, fewer meals.

Why?

Because when people ate only 2 – 3 meals per day, they found it very hard to control their calories due to hunger, which led to overeating. By eating 4 – 6 meals per day, however, people found it much easier to stick to their diet plans because they never felt famished.

So, while some people have figured out how to make 2 – 3 large meals per day work in terms of fat loss and muscle growth, I've found that method of dieting significantly harder to stick to than 4 – 6 smaller meals per day.

THE THIRD LAW OF FAT LOSS:
USE CARDIO TO HELP BURN FAT

As you know, doing cardio doesn't equal burning fat. It can accelerate fat loss by burning calories and by speeding up your metabolic rate, but whether you actually lose fat or not will be determined by your daily caloric intake and expenditure.

Now, with that being said, most guys find cardio necessary in order to get into the "super lean" category (10% body fat and under) because you can only cut your calories so much before you start to lose strength and muscle mass. Some, however, don't need to bother—they simply regulate their calories and get as lean as they want. This is really just a matter of genetics and individual physiology.

THE BOTTOM LINE

Believe it or not, easy fat loss depends on these three laws and no others. The U.S. weight loss market generates over *$60 billion per year*, and, drugs and invasive surgeries aside, any and all workable weight loss methods rely on the three simple rules you just read to achieve results.

Sure, you can get fancy and count "points" instead of calories, can come up with all kinds of creative recipes, can have your miniature desserts, and so on. Regardless, the fundamentals of fat loss don't need a fancy name or marketing campaign. They really are this simple.

3

HOW TO EAT RIGHT WITHOUT OBSESSING OVER EVERY CALORIE

I HAVE GOOD NEWS.

You can look and feel great without breaking out a calculator every time you eat.

Getting proper nutrition is a precise science, but it doesn't have to be agonizing. In fact, I recommend a more laid-back approach. If you make planning or tracking meals too complicated, you'll have trouble sticking with it.

That being said, in order to lose fat, you must keep your body burning more energy than you're feeding it, and the energy potential of food is measured in calories. Eat too many calories—give your body more potential energy than it needs—and it has no incentive to burn fat.

In order to gain muscle, your body needs a surplus of energy to repair and rebuild itself (along with plenty of protein). Thus, you need to eat slightly more than your body burns to get bigger.

In this chapter I'm going to share some simple rules that you can follow to eat right. Just by following these rules, you'll find that you can lose or gain weight when you want to and that you'll feel healthy and vital.

1. MAKE SURE YOU EAT ENOUGH

A calorie is a measurement of the potential energy found in food, and your body burns quite a bit of energy every day. Everything from the beating of your heart to the digestion of your food requires energy, and your body has to get it from the food you eat.

Thus, it's important that you feed your body enough, and that's especially true when you work out. If you underfeed your body, don't be surprised if you don't have the energy to train hard or if you feel generally exhausted.

- Eat 1 gram of protein per pound of body weight per day.

- Eat 1.5 grams of carbs per pound of body weight per day.

- Eat 1 gram of healthy fats per 4 pounds of body weight per day.

That's where you start. For a 200 lb male, it would look like this:

- 200 grams of protein per day

- 300 grams of carbs per day

- 50 grams of fat per day

That's about 2,500 calories per day, which should work for making slow, steady muscle and strength gains without any fat added along the way (which really should be the goal of "maintenance"—not staying the exact same).

If your priority is to gain muscle, then you need to add about 500 calories per day to your "maintenance" diet. The easiest way to do this is to bump up your carbs by about 50 grams per day, and your fats by about 30 grams per day.

If you're trying to lose fat, then you need to subtract about 500 calories per day from your maintenance diet. To do this, drop your carbs by about 100 grams per day and your fats by about 10 grams per day.

It's also important that you consume high-quality calories. Junk food calories, such as white bread and pastas, chips, and juice and soda, will make you look and feel like crap, while good calories, such as fruits, vegetables, whole grains, and lean proteins, will keep you in tip-top shape.

2. EAT ENOUGH PROTEIN

If you work out, you need more protein than someone who doesn't work out. Why? Because exercise causes muscle damage.

With every rep you perform, you're causing "micro-tears" in your muscle fibers, and your body needs protein to fully repair this damage. The body doesn't just repair them to their previous state, however; it builds them bigger and stronger so it can better handle the stress of exercise.

So, in order to get the most out of your workouts, you need to eat enough protein. And that doesn't mean just eating a lot after working out.

It means eating enough every day, which will require you to eat some with every meal you have (and as a general rule, eating .75-1 gram of protein per pound of body weight is a good target if you exercise regularly).

By doing this, you can ensure your body has the amino acids it needs to build muscle and repair tissue. If you fail to feed your body enough protein, it will fall behind in the muscle breakdown and repair cycle, and you can actually get smaller and weaker despite exercise.

There are two main sources of protein out there: whole food protein and supplement protein.

Whole food protein is, as you guessed, protein that comes from natural food sources, such as beef, chicken, fish, etc. The best forms of whole food protein are chicken, turkey, lean red meat, fish, eggs, and milk.

If you're vegetarian, your best options are eggs, low-fat cottage cheese (Organic Valley is my favorite brand), low-fat European style (Greek) yogurt (0% Fage is my favorite), tempeh, tofu, quinoa, almonds, rice, and beans.

While we're on the subject of vegetarianism, some people claim that you must carefully combine your proteins if you're vegetarian or vegan to ensure your body is getting "complete" proteins (all of the amino acids needed to build tissue). This theory and the faulty research it was based on was thoroughly debunked as a myth by the American Dietetic Association, yet it still hangs around. While it's true that some sources of vegetable protein are lower in certain amino acids than other forms of protein, there is no scientific evidence to prove that they lack them altogether.

Protein supplements are powdered or liquid foods that contain protein from various sources, such as whey (a liquid remaining after milk has been curdled and strained in the process of making cheese), egg, and soy—the three most common sources of supplement protein. There are also great plant-based supplements out there that are a blend of high-quality protein sources such as quinoa, brown rice, peas, hemp, and fruit.

You don't NEED protein supplements to eat well, but it can be impractical for some to try to get all protein from whole foods considering the fact that you will be eating protein 4 – 6 times per day.

Now, there are a few things you should know about eating protein. First is the subject of how much protein you can absorb in one sitting. Studies relating to this are very contradictory and disputed, mainly because it's a complex subject. Your genetics, metabolism, digestive tract health, lifestyle, and amount of lean mass are all important factors. But in the spirit of keeping things simple, here's what we know: you can eat and properly use a lot of protein in each meal. How much, exactly? Well, your body should have no trouble absorbing upwards of 100 grams in one sitting.

That said, there aren't any benefits of eating this way (I find gorging quite uncomfortable, actually), but it's good to know in case you miss a meal and need to make it up by loading protein into a later meal.

Another thing to know about protein is that different proteins digest at different speeds, and some are better utilized by the body than others. Beef protein, for example, is digested quickly, and 70 – 80% of what's eaten is utilized by the body (the exact number varies based on what study you read, but they all fall between 70 – 80%). Whey protein is also digested quickly and its "net protein utilization" (NPU) is in the low 90% range. Egg protein digests much slower than whey and beef, and its NPU also falls in the same range.

NPU and digestion speeds are important to know because you want to rely on high-NPU proteins to meet your daily protein requirement, and you want a quick-digesting protein for your post-workout meal, and a slow-digesting protein for your final meal before you go to bed (to help you get through the fasting that occurs during sleep).

I could give you charts and tables of the NPU rates of various proteins, but I'm going to just keep it simple. In order to meet your daily protein requirements, here are your choices:

Whole Food Proteins

Lean meats (beef, pork, chicken, and turkey)

Fish

Eggs

Vegetarian sources noted above

Protein Supplements

Egg

Whey

Casein

High-quality plant-based protein supplements

These are all considered "complete proteins," meaning they contain all of the essential amino acids for cellular repair and growth that your body can't synthesize itself (it creates some and has to get the rest from food).

In case you're wondering why I left soy protein off the list of recommended supplements, it's because it's just a bad protein source. To start, most soy protein supplements use genetically modified soybeans (which is a very dangerous trend encroaching further and further into the world of agriculture), and studies have shown that too much of it can increase estrogen levels and inhibit your body's testosterone production (due to a plant estrogen found in soybeans). Just stay away from it.

3. EAT HEALTHY FATS

Fats are the densest energy source available to your body. Each gram of fat contains over twice the calories of a gram of carbohydrate or protein. Healthy fats, such as those found in olive oil, avocados, flax seed oil, many nuts, and other foods, are actually an important component for overall good health. Fats help your body absorb the other nutrients that you give it; they nourish the nervous system, help maintain cell structures, regulate hormone levels, and more.

Saturated fats are a form of fat found mainly in animal products such as meat, dairy products, and egg yolks. Some plant foods, such as coconut oil, palm oil, and palm kernel oil, are also high in saturated fats. While it's commonly believed that eating saturated fat harms your health, the opposite is actually true. Recent studies have shown that including saturated fats in your diet can reduce your risk of heart disease.

Trans fats are scientifically modified saturated fats that have been engineered to give foods longer shelf lives. Many cheap, packaged foods are full of trans fats (such as run-of-the-mill popcorn, yogurt, and peanut butter) as are many frozen foods (such as frozen pizza, packaged pastries, cakes, etc.). And fried foods are often fried in trans fats. These fats are bad news, and eating too much of them can lead to all kinds of diseases and complications. They have no nutritional value for the body and thus should be avoided altogether.

Most people eat more fat than is necessary, thus adding lots of unnecessary calories to their daily intake. Getting enough healthy fats every day is pretty simple. Here's how it works:

- Keep your intake of saturated fats relatively low (below 10% of your total calories). Saturated fat is found in foods like meat, dairy products, eggs, coconut oil, bacon fat, and lard. If a fat is solid at room temperature, it's a saturated fat.

- Completely avoid trans fats. Trans fats are found in processed foods such as cookies, cakes, fries, and doughnuts. Any food that contains "hydrogenated oil" or "partially hydrogenated oil" likely contains trans fats, so just don't eat it. (Sure, having a cheat here and there that contains trans fats won't harm anything, but you definitely don't want to eat them regularly.)

- Get at least half of your daily fat from unsaturated fats such as olive oil, nuts, peanut oil, avocados, flax seed oil, safflower oil, or sesame oil. If a fat is liquid at room temperature, it's an unsaturated fat.

4. EAT GOOD CARBS

The carbohydrate is probably the most misunderstood, maligned, and feared macro-nutrient. Thanks to the scores of bogus diet plans and suggestions out there, many people equate eating carbs with getting fat. While eating TOO MANY carbs can make you fat (just as eating too much protein or fat can), carbs are hardly your enemy. They play an essential role in not only muscle growth but in overall body function.

Regardless of what type of carbohydrate you eat—broccoli or apple pie—the body breaks it down into two substances: *glucose* and *glycogen*. Glucose is commonly referred to as "blood sugar," and it's an energy source used by your cells to do the many things they do. Glycogen is a substance stored in the liver and muscles that can be easily converted to glucose for immediate energy. When you lift weights intensely, your muscles burn up their glycogen stores to cope with the overload.

Now, why is broccoli good for you but apple pie isn't? Because your body reacts very differently to broccoli than to apple pie. You've probably heard the terms "simple" and "complex" carbs before and wondered what they meant. You might have also heard of the *glycemic index* and wondered what it was all about.

These things are actually pretty simple. The glycemic index is a numeric system of ranking how quickly carbohydrates are converted into glucose in the body. Carbs are ranked on a scale of 0 to 100 depending how they affect blood sugar levels once eaten. A GI rating of 55 and under is considered "low GI," 56 to 69 is medium, and 70 and above is high on the index. A "simple" carb is one that converts very quickly (is high on the glycemic index), such as table sugar, honey, and watermelon, while a "complex" carb is one that converts slowly (is low on the glycemic index), such as broccoli, apple, and whole-grain bread.

It's very important to know where the carbs you eat fall on the index, because studies have linked regular consumption of high-GI carbs to increased risk for heart disease, diabetes, and obesity.

The amount of carbohydrates that you should eat every day depends on what you're trying to accomplish. Building muscle requires that you eat a substantial amount of carbs, while dieting to lose weight requires that you reduce carbs.

Regardless of how many carbs you need to eat per day, there's a simple rule to follow regarding high-, medium- and low-glycemic carbs.

Eat carbs in the medium–high range of the glycemic index (70 – 90 is a good rule of thumb) about 30 minutes before you exercise, and again within 30 minutes of finishing your workout.

The reason you want some carbs before training is that you need the energy for your training. The reason you want them after is that your muscles' glycogen stores are heavily depleted, and by replacing it quickly, you actually help your body maintain an anabolic state and not lose muscle tissue.

My favorite pre- and post-workout carbs are bananas and rice milk, but other good choices are baked potato, instant oatmeal, and fruits that are above 60 on the glycemic index, such as cantaloupe, pineapple, watermelon, dates, apricots, and figs. Some people recommend eating foods high in table sugar (sucrose) after working out because it's high on the GI, but I stay away from processed sugar as much as possible.

All other carbs you eat should be in the middle or at the low end of the glycemic index (60 and below is a good rule of thumb). It really is that simple. If you follow this rule, you'll avoid so many problems that others suffer from due to the energy highs and lows that come with eating high-GI carbs that burn the body out.

Below is a list of common snack foods with corresponding average GI scores. The GI scores vary a bit from brand to brand, but not by much. Generally speaking, it's best to stay away from these types of carbs.

(The following information is sourced from the University of Sydney, the University of Harvard, and Livestrong.com.)

FOOD	GI
White bread bagel	72
Corn chips	63
Pretzels	83
Candy bar	62-78
Wheat or corn cracker	67-87

Rye cracker	64
Rice cake	78
Popcorn	72
White rice	64
Pizza	80
Raisins	64
Whole wheat bread	71
White bread	70
Baguette	95
English muffin (white bread)	77
Baked potato	85
Muesli	66

So, forget stuff like sugar, white bread, processed, low-quality whole wheat bread, bagels, junk cereals, muffins, white pasta, crackers, waffles, rice cakes, corn flakes, and white rice. I wouldn't even recommend eating these things often as pre- or post-workout carbs because they're just not good for your body.

Even certain fruits, such as watermelon and dates, are bad snack foods because of where they fall on the glycemic index. If you're unsure about a carb you like, look it up to see where it falls on the glycemic index. If it's above 60, just leave it out of your meals that aren't immediately before or after working out.

5. EAT YOUR FRUITS AND VEGGIES

Your body requires many different things to function optimally. It can't look and feel great on protein and carbs alone. You need calcium to ensure your muscles can contract and relax properly. You need fiber to help move food through the digestive tract. You need iron to carry oxygen to your cells and create energy.

There are many other "little helpers" that your body needs to perform its many physiological processes, and fruits and vegetables contain many vital nutrients that you can't get from vitamin supplements. By eating 3 – 5 servings of both fruits and vegetables per day, you enjoy the many benefits that these nutrients give to your body, such as lowering your risk of cancer, heart disease, diabetes, and many other diseases.

This isn't hard to do, either. A medium-sized piece of fruit is one serving, as is half a cup of berries. A cup of greens is a serving of vegetables, as is half a cup of other vegetables.

Fruit juices, however, are another story. While they may seem like an easy way to get in your daily fruits, they are actually not much more than tasty sugar water. Not only do most fruit juices have sugar added, but the juice has also been separated from the fruit's fibrous pulp, which slows down the metabolism of the sugars. Without that, the juice becomes a very high-glycemic drink. You're better off drinking water and eating whole fruit.

The exception to this is creating juice using a juicer or blender to grind up the entire piece of fruit, removing nothing. This, of course, is no different than chewing up the fruit in your mouth.

Fruits widely recognized as the healthiest are apples, bananas, blueberries, oranges, grapefruit, strawberries, and pineapples.

Vegetables often recommended as the healthiest are asparagus, broccoli, spinach, sweet potatoes, tomatoes, carrots, onions, and eggplant.

6. PLAN AND PROPORTION YOUR MEALS PROPERLY

Many people's meal plans are engineered for getting fat. They skip breakfast, eat a junk food lunch, come home famished, have a big dinner with some dessert, and then have a snack like chips or popcorn while watching TV at night.

A much better strategy is to eat smaller meals every 3-4 hours, and include protein with each (as this fills you up and makes you feel satisfied).

Much of your daily carbohydrates should come before and after training, when your body needs them most. I eat about 10 – 15% of my daily carbs before training, and about 30 – 40% after, in my post-workout meal.

It's also important when dieting to lose weight to not eat carbs within several hours of going to bed. This advice has been kicking around the health and fitness world for quite some time, but usually with the wrong explanation.

There's no scientific evidence that eating carbs at night or before bed will lead to gaining fat, but it can *hinder* fat loss. How?

The insulin created by the body to process and absorb carbs eaten stops the use of fat as an energy source. Your body naturally burns the most fat while sleeping, and so going to sleep with elevated insulin levels interferes with fat loss.

Related to this is the fact that studies have indicated that the production and processing of insulin interferes with the production and processing of growth hormone, which has powerful fat-burning properties. Your body naturally produces much of its growth hormone while sleeping, so again, if your body is flushed with insulin when you go to sleep, your growth hormone production may suffer, which in turn may rob you of its fat-burning and muscle-building benefits.

So, as a general rule, when you're dieting to lose weight, don't eat any carbs within 4 – 5 hours of bedtime. You should only consume lean proteins after dinner. I follow this rule when bulking too, not because I'm worried about fat burning (you don't burn fat when bulking), but because I don't want to stunt my growth hormone production.

You can spread your fats throughout the day. I like to start my day with 1 – 2 tablespoons of a 3-6-9 blend, but you don't have to get one if you don't want to. You can simply stick to the sources of healthy fat given earlier.

7. DRINK A LOT OF WATER

The human body is about 60% water in adult males and about 70% in adult females. Muscles are about 70% water. That alone tells you how important staying hydrated is to maintaining good health and proper body function. Your body's ability to digest, transport, and absorb nutrients from food is dependent upon proper fluid intake. Water helps prevent injuries in the gym by cushioning joints and other soft-tissue areas. When your body is dehydrated, literally every physiological process is negatively affected.

I really can't stress enough the importance of drinking clean, pure water. It has zero calories, so it will never cause you to gain weight regardless of how much you drink. (You can actually harm your body by drinking too much water, but this would require that you drink several gallons per day.)

The Institute of Medicine reported in 2004 that women should consume about 91 ounces of water—or three-quarters of a gallon—per day, and men should consume about 125 ounces per day (a gallon is 128 ounces).

Now, keep in mind that those numbers include the water found in food. The average person gets about 80% of their water from drinking it and other beverages, and about 20% from the food they eat.

I've been drinking 1 – 2 gallons of water per day for years now, which is more than the IOM baseline recommendation, but I sweat a fair amount due to exercise and I live in Florida, which surely makes my needs higher. I fill a one-gallon jug at the start of my day and simply make sure that I finish it by dinner time. By the time I go to bed, I'll have drank a few more glasses.

Make sure the water you drink is filtered, purified water and not tap water (disgusting, but some people drink it). There's a big difference between drinking clean, alkaline water that your body can fully utilize and drinking polluted, acidic junk from the tap or bottle (which is the case with certain brands such as Dasani and Aquafina).

8. CUT BACK ON THE SODIUM

The average American's diet is so over-saturated with sodium it makes my head spin.

The Institute of Medicine recommends 1,500 milligrams of sodium per day as the adequate intake level for most adults. According to the CDC, the average American aged 2 and up eats *3,436 milligrams* of sodium per day.

Too much sodium in the body causes water retention (which gives you that puffy, soft look) and it can lead to high blood pressure and heart disease.

Frozen and canned foods are full of sodium, as are cured meats like bacon and sausage (one slice of bacon contains *1,000 milligrams* of sodium!).

When you need to add salt to your food,, I recommend sea salt or Himalayan rock salt (sounds like fancy BS, but it's actually great stuff) because it has many naturally occurring minerals, whereas run-of-the-mill table salt has been "chemically cleaned" to remove "impurities," which includes these vital elements.

9. CHEAT CORRECTLY

Many people struggling with diets talk about "cheat days." The idea is that if you're good during the week, you can go buck wild on the weekends and somehow not gain fat. Well, unless you have a very fast metabolism, that's not how it works. If you follow a strict diet and exercise, you can expect to lose 1 – 2 pounds per week. If you get too crazy, you can gain it right back over a weekend.

So don't think cheat DAYS, think cheat MEALS—meals where you eat more or less anything you want (and all other meals of the week follow your meal plan). When done once or twice per week, a cheat meal is not only satisfying, but it can actually help you lose fat.

How?

Well, first there's the psychological boost, which keeps you happy and motivated, which ultimately makes sticking to your diet easier.

But there's also a physiological boost.

Studies on overfeeding (the scientific term for binging on food) show that doing so can boost your metabolic rate by anywhere from 3-10%.

While this sounds good, it actually doesn't mean much when you consider that you would need to eat anywhere from a few hundred to a few thousand extra calories in a day to achieve this effect.

More important are the effects cheating has on a hormone called leptin, which regulates hunger, your metabolic rate, appetite, motivation, and libido, as well as serving other functions in your body.

When you're in a caloric deficit and lose body fat, your leptin levels drop. This, in turn, causes your metabolism to slow down, your appetite to increase, your motivation to wane, and your mood to sour.

On the other hand, when you give your body more energy (calories) than it needs, leptin levels are boosted, which can then have positive effects on fat oxidation, thyroid activity, mood, and even testosterone levels.

So if it's a leptin boost that you really want, how do you best achieve it?

Eating carbohydrates is the most effective way. Second to that is eating protein (high-protein meals also raise your metabolic rate). Dietary fats aren't very effective at increasing leptin levels, and alcohol actually inhibits it.

So, if your weight is stuck and you're irritable and demotivated, a nice kick of leptin might be all you need to get the scales moving again.

Have a nice cheat meal full of protein and carbs, and feel good about it.

(I would recommend, however, that you don't go too overboard with your cheat meals—don't eat 2,000 calories of junk food and desserts and think it won't do anything.)

THE BOTTOM LINE

You may find this chapter a bit hard to swallow (no pun intended). Some people have a really hard time giving up their unhealthy eating habits (sugar and junk food can be pretty addictive). That being said, consider the following benefits of following the advice in this chapter:

1. If this is a completely new way of eating for you, I *guarantee* you'll feel better than you have in a *long* time. You won't have energy highs and lows. You won't feel lethargic. You won't have that mental fogginess that comes with being stuffed full of unhealthy food every day.

2. You will appreciate "bad" food so much more when you only have it once or twice per week. You'd be surprised how much better a dessert tastes when you haven't had one in a week. (You may also be surprised that junk food that you loved in the past no longer tastes good.)

3. You will actually come to enjoy healthy foods. I *promise*. Even if they don't taste good to you at first, just groove in the routine, and soon you'll crave brown rice and fruit instead of doughnuts and bread. Your body will adapt.

This chapter teaches you all there really is to eating properly so you can build muscle or lose weight on demand, all while staying healthy.

Now that we've looked at what it takes to lose fat, and what role cardio plays in it, let's get to the workouts themselves!

4

FAT INCINERATING CARDIO CIRCUIT

CALORIES BURNED:

550–800 per hour

GOING TO THE GYM AND HITTING up the cardio equipment day after day after day is going to get incredibly boring, incredibly fast. That's why you need a new game plan. You need a form of cardio that's constantly changing, never allowing you a chance to get bored.

In addition to that, you also need a form of cardio that will not only burn calories while you are doing it, but also causes the body to continue to burn calories for hours after it's completed.

That's precisely what the fat-incinerating cardio circuit is going to do. This circuit is going to combine a mixture of movements that keep your heart rate up, keep your body moving, and make sure that you see nothing but top-notch fat-loss benefits.

Another nice thing about cardio circuit training is that it can double up as strength training if you use enough weight for it to be a muscular challenge.

To do the fat-incinerating cardio circuit, you're going to select from a number of different exercises that target all the main muscle groups in the body. Do your best to choose dumbbell or bodyweight exercises only, as this will reduce your chances of standing around waiting for gym equipment to open up. Furthermore, it also makes it possible to complete the workouts in the comfort of your own home if desired.

Once you have your exercises set, then you're going to perform 10–15 reps of each exercise, without stopping, and then move directly to the next exercise.

A good way to set up the structure of this workout program is to perform one lower-body exercise, one upper-body exercise, and then either one cardio conditioning exercise or one abdominal exercise, for one minute.

This will ensure that your entire body gets worked evenly, while also helping to prevent the buildup of a large amount of fatigue. Since the lower body can rest while you're doing your upper-body exercise, and vice versa, this will enable you to keep up the pace required for this workout session.

Aim to complete a total of 12 exercises in a row, and then rest for two or three minutes before repeating again. How many rounds of this you do will depend on your fitness level, but aim for somewhere between two and five for best results.

Here is a sample circuit that you could perform:

- Dumbbell Squats

- Dumbbell Floor Chest Press

- Jumping Jacks

- Dumbbell Lunges

- Dumbbell Shoulder Press

- Burpees

- Dumbbell Deadlift

- Dumbbell Bent-Over Row

- Plank

- Dumbbell Step-Ups

- Dumbbell T Raises

- Jump Roping

Get creative and come up with a circuit that works the areas of your body that you want to improve most.

5

STAIR SPRINTS

CALORIES BURNED:

550 – 700 per hour

WANT A FIRMER BACKSIDE? MORE powerful thighs? Want to burn fat like never before? If so, Stair Sprints, also sometimes referred to as "Tower Running," are an excellent exercise choice.

This workout session will be just as intense, if not more intense, than a very fast-paced run. The main muscles that you'll be hitting each time you launch up the stairs for another sprint will include the glutes, hamstrings, squads, calves, as well as all the muscles in the core and those running along the spinal column.

If your calves are slow to respond to training, this cardio variety is going to change that dramatically. Since your calf muscles engage with every step, this form of cardio will definitely get them reacting and growing noticeably more defined.

So, what does Stair Sprinting consist of?

Find a very long staircase somewhere (10–15 floors is plenty to start with). This could be an apartment building, an office building (preferably one that isn't all that populated and be sure to check ahead of time for permission to use it). You could find stairs outside as well, such as those in a sports stadium.

Start at the bottom of the stairs and, once ready, run as fast as you can to the top. Once you reach the top, simply walk back down, using this as your rest period for the interval session.

Once you're able to do this 10–15 times consecutively (depending on how long the staircase is), you'll want to start adding some advanced variations into the mix.

Try going up the staircase using only one leg. Once at the top, come back down and then reverse it, so you're using the other leg. This is an incredible strength builder, and is quite tough—don't be surprised if you need to stop and rest halfway up when you first get started.

Another variation is double jumps. Try taking two stairs at a time rather than just one. This increased stride is going to help target the hamstrings more.

Finally, if you want something really different, consider going up sideways or, if you're really skilled, backwards. Just be sure to have someone watching out for you and try and take note of others around you before you start going up the staircase.

Stair sprints are a fantastic way to tone and firm up your lower body, while helping you get into the best cardiovascular shape of your life. Give them a try next time you're heading for a cardio workout and need something fresh and challenging.

6

BOX YOUR WAY INTO SHAPE

CALORIES BURNED:

400 – 550 per hour

ONE OF THE BEST WAYS TO build up your upper-body strength and muscular endurance while burning off a very high amount of calories is boxing. More and more people are taking up boxing as a form of cardio activity, and if you've never thought of this one before, why not give it a shot?

Boxing is a fantastic way to stay in shape, have some fun, and achieve a desirable body composition. This form of exercise is going to help increase your overall cardiovascular capacity, improve your muscular endurance, as well as help build up your speed and quickness, especially in the upper body.

If you happen to be participating in any sports that require you to have a faster reaction time, this can be hugely advantageous.

If you've never boxed before, it may be a good idea to look into taking some introductory lessons, just so you can learn proper punching technique and all the different variations that you can do as you go about your boxing workout. This will ensure that you stay injury free and achieve the greatest overall benefits from your workouts.

After you've learned all the basic boxing moves, you will have a few different options for structuring your workout program.

First, consider performing just one punch for one minute, then switch to another punch for another minute. Continue repeating this process, either using different types of punches, depending on your skill level, or going back and forth between a few, until 5–10 minutes has passed.

Then stop and walk around the room for five minutes before going in for a second round.

Another way to structure the workout is to combine a mixture of punches into a sequence. This is likely what you'll do as you move to a higher level of boxing skill, and what you will be doing if you ever choose to participate in boxing classes.

Because stringing together combinations of punches requires that you constantly change direction and movement patterns, you'll definitely notice improvements in agility and mind-muscle coordination.

Keep in mind that you should never keep your feet completely stationary and locked to the ground. Maintain a light bounce to your step patterns so that you get the lower body working too and further bump up your heart rate.

Finally, consider listening to some fast-paced music while doing your boxing workout. This can definitely help to increase the amount of energy you give to the session, boosting your calorie burn.

So, give your lower body a rest from the traditional cardio sessions you're doing and give your upper body a chance to shine. Boxing is a perfect way to burn fat fast and add more variety to your workout program.

7

HIGH INTENSITY INTERVAL TRAINING (HIIT)

<u>CALORIES BURNED:</u>

450 – 650 calories per hour

YOU'VE LIKELY HEARD OF "sprint" training or "interval" training and maybe wondered if this is something you should be doing or not. Well, the short answer is *absolutely*.

Why? Because it's been scientifically proven to burn more fat than traditional, "steady state" cardio (where you maintain a steady level of exertion)—and it takes less time!

So, how does it work? The HIIT method involves doing a cardio activity, such as running, biking, or swimming, as hard as you can for 20–60 seconds, and then backing down to a low-intensity rest for two or three minutes, followed by a high-intensity burst, and so on.

These intervals are carefully timed and you generally do 6–10 rounds per session, starting with a five-minute warm-up, and ending with a five-minute cool-down. Your goal should be to work up to 25–30 minutes of HIIT, which is quite a workout.

If you're new to HIIT, I recommend that you ease into it at your own pace. Don't worry about being super strict on your timing. If you wanted to sprint for 30 seconds but can only make it for 20 before feeling like your legs are going to give in, stop there. If you need four minutes for your heart rate to come back down, take four minutes.

You can even forget the timing altogether at first. Once you're warmed up and ready to start, you can do the high-intensity interval for as long as your body can go before it says "enough!" Then slow down to a brisk walk or jog, depending on what you're capable of, and take as much time as you need before moving to the next high-intensity interval.

HIIT is hands down one of the most effective forms of cardio out there, so I highly recommend that you include at least one HIIT session per week among your other cardio workouts (but feel free to do more if you're up to it!).

8

BURN MORE CALORIES WITH LATERAL BOUNDS

CALORIES BURNED:

700 – 1100 per hour

LATERAL BOUNDS ARE PERFECT for those who want to blast fat fast because they burn up many hundreds of calories per hour, and help to firm and tone all the major lower-body muscles, as well as your core. In addition to that, they're perfect for those who are participating in athletic activities because they'll also help to improve your agility and balance.

Here's how to do them: Start by standing on your right leg. Bend down a little bit to engage your quads. Jump laterally to your left, and land on your left foot. Bend down a little again, now on your other leg. Jump back to your right foot. This completes one repetition.

If you would like to add even more of a challenge to your lateral bounds, try tapping one hand on the floor with each bound you make. To do so, as soon as you land on the ground after each bound, bend over at the waist and place one hand on the floor in front of you. This will not only burn more calories, but also engage your ab muscles.

For workout design purposes, you'll want to start by aiming for between two and four bounds in a row, without a rest. Use this time to really get a good feel for the movement pattern and make sure that you are using good form.

Once you're comfortable, increase it to 10 bounds at a time before resting. Aim for three sets of 10 per session. After you can do that easily, bump it up to 20. That'll really get your heart racing and the calories burning.

Continue adding increments of 10 bounds, performing three sets total each workout until you're up to doing 50 bounds per set. When that becomes too easy for you, increase the total sets to keep yourself challenged.

9

CREATE A MINI-
TRIATHLON

CALORIES BURNED:

500 – 700 per hour

THE GREAT THING ABOUT incorporating a number of different cardio methods into each workout session that you perform is the fact that you'll work more groups of muscles. If all you do is bike day after day after day, your quads and hamstrings might become incredibly conditioned, but the rest of your body will be neglected.

So, to create your mini-triathlon, you'll first want to select three different modes of cardio training that you'd like to do. The real triathlon events utilize running, swimming, and cycling, but do not feel like you have to stick with these.

If you'd prefer to add the cross-trainer into the mix, so be it. Rowing is also another excellent form of cardio, and if you have a rowing machine at your gym, you should definitely be making good use of it. Jump roping is another excellent form of cardio to consider.

Once you do have your forms of cardio selected, designate a certain time frame to each. Again, realize that you don't necessarily have to spend the same amount of time with each exercise.

Jump roping, for example, is highly intense, so chances are you wouldn't do it for 20 minutes straight; you may only jump rope for 10 minutes, and then move on to biking, jogging, uphill walking, or whatever other form of cardio you've decided to include.

For this workout session, since you won't be incorporating any interval training or other incredibly intense techniques into the session, aim for no less than 30 minutes total between your three chosen forms of activity.

After you complete each style of cardio, you can stop for a few minutes to perform some light stretching and catch your breath if necessary, but avoid sitting around, as this will cause you to lose momentum and intensity.

10

SUPERSETS FOR SUPER FAT LOSS

CALORIES BURNED:

450–500 per hour

NO TIME TO GET INTO THE gym to perform a cardio and strength training workout? If you're like most people, you lead a busy life. Aiming for the traditional three or four days per week and between two and four additional days of cardio training may be just a little too much for you to handle with all that you have going on.

Does this mean you have to forget about getting into shape and losing fat?

Not a chance.

You simply need a fast, effective program that will help you burn fat and improve strength and muscle tone. Well, that's precisely what this cardio method is.

The idea behind superset training is that you do two strength moves back-to-back, with no rest in between. Supersets keep your heart rate elevated and have similar effects as an interval training session because you'll be exercising hard for about a minute (30 seconds for each set) and then resting for a minute before you start your next superset.

When selecting the exercises to pair in your supersets, I recommend that you stick to compound movements (exercises that engage multiple muscle groups, such as the squat, bench press, deadlift, pull-ups, etc.)

The more muscle groups you can work with any specific exercise, the more calories you'll burn.

Now, to build your superset routine, choose five or six exercises that work your upper and lower body and your core, and ensure you include a few compound exercises. You'll then want to do 10–15 repetitions per exercise and go through the list twice.

That should give you a 20–25 minute workout session to perform three times per week (one day off between sessions), which is something that even the busiest person should be able to handle.

Here's a sample routine to get you started:

Superset #1:

Squat

Shoulder Press

Superset #2:

Deadlift

Bench Press

Superset #3:

Lunge

Bent-Over Row

Superset #4:

Step-Up

Pull-Up

Superset #5:

Plank

Cable Crunch

11

DANCE THE FAT
AWAY WITH ZUMBA

CALORIES BURNED:

300 – 500 per hour

ONE OF THE LATEST FITNESS "crazes" to hit the mainstream market is Zumba dancing. Tons of people have flocked to this new style of exercise, and for a good reason—it works! Zumba workouts are a fun way to get your heart rate up, improve your balance and agility, and firm and strengthen your lower body and core.

Zumba originated back in 2001 when fitness trainer Beto Perez came across the concept of Latin dance and turned this into a workout sensation. Since then, it's been brought into North America and has rapidly caught on, with classes regularly held in just about every major city that you can name. Zumba is not just a workout for women, either. Men of all ages are enjoying it as a major part of their workout routines.

A nice thing about Zumba is that it's very low-impact, giving your joints a nice break from any other rigorous activities that you might be doing throughout the week. Since this workout is performed to Latin music, it's also going to improve your sense of rhythm and coordination.

When you first look into Zumba classes, you'll likely find that there are many different options available. Let's look at these more closely.

BEGINNER AND ADVANCED ZUMBA

The beginner classes are great introductions to this form of cardio workout. In them, you learn the basic movements at a slower pace, while the advanced classes keep you moving continuously throughout the workout at a higher intensity.

ZUMBA TONING

If you're looking to focus on firming and toning your muscles, these classes are for you. Zumba Toning classes challenge your muscular strength more than others, hitting the abs, legs, and the upper body. All of the strength moves are still completed in rhythm with the music, so you won't lose the feel of the Zumba workout.

ZUMBA IN THE CIRCUIT

Zumba in the Circuit is a style of Zumba exercise that uses a circuit training routine, moving from one exercise to another. Like Zumba Toning classes, the circuit routines build overall body strength more than regular classes, and they also burn a higher amount of calories.

AQUA ZUMBA

Finally, for those who want something completely different, Aqua Zumba takes the workout into the water. Since you'll be working against the resistance of the water, you'll still see excellent conditioning benefits from this style of class with no impact. It's a fun change!

12

BURN FAT FAST WITH TABATA TRAINING

CALORIES BURNED:

300 – 400 per 20 minutes

AFTER SETTING THE GOAL that you're going to try and burn off fat as quickly as you possibly can, the second step is figuring out a workout program that's going to allow you to do just that.

Enter Tabata training. This cardio method was invented by Dr. Izumi Tabata at the National Institute of Fitness and Sports in Tokyo. This interval training hybrid workout is the king of calorie burn. Not only will you burn a chunk of calories while you do it, but you will also burn many more for days after the workout is completed. (Yes, you read correctly—days. To be specific, for up to two days according to a study done by Laval University in Quebec.)

So how do you do this killer workout?

What you do is perform 20 seconds of full-out, maximum effort exercise and then stop and rest for 10 seconds immediately after. Once the 10-second rest is up, you jump right back into full exertion. You do this eight times before stopping to rest for two to three minutes.

If you aren't gasping for air after just your first four-minute routine, you probably weren't working hard enough!

Make sure that you get have a stopwatch for this style of training because keeping the timing precise is an important part of reaping its full benefits.

Now, which exercises should you be doing during the Tabata workout?

I recommend that you choose movements that work as many muscle groups as possible. The more muscles you work, the more calories you burn, and the more toned you get.

Don't be afraid to do traditional weight lifting movements (but do them with low weight, of course!). These can work perfectly for Tabata training, and since you're only performing them for 20 seconds at a time, you should be able to maintain proper form.

Just be sure that you lighten the weight considerably as this is a cardio workout, not a strength one.

Some of the top moves to consider are:

- Squats

- Squat to press

- Deadlift

- Clean and jerk

- Burpees

- Mountain climbers

- Jump roping

- Uphill running sprints

Always rest for two or three minutes between each four-minute training period to allow the body to recover. In the beginning, you'll probably find it too hard to do more than two or three of the four-minute blasts—that's plenty to start with. As you improve, try to work up to four training periods (still with two or three minutes of rest between each).

If you're running really short on time and can only perform a single four-minute round, don't fret—those four minutes can still be an incredibly effective workout.

Tabata is one of the most effective fat-burning forms of cardio that you can do. And if you're short on time, it simply can't be beaten.

13

GET FIT BY PLAYING VIDEO GAMES

CALORIES BURNED:

350 – 600 per hour

WHEN YOU THINK OF VIDEO games, you hardly think of getting in shape. On the contrary, you probably think of moving nothing but your thumbs for hours on end, eyes transfixed to the screen.

Times are changing, though. Video gaming isn't just about going catatonic on the couch. There are now video games that get you up, moving around, interacting with the game and doing exercise! They are currently made for the Wii and Xbox because these consoles have devices that can track your movements and thus allow your body movements to affect the game.

Examples of these games are Wii Fit, Gold's Gym Dance Workout, Active, and The Biggest Loser Challenge. These games offer quite a variety of ways to burn calories. Whether you want to improve your golf game, go for a downhill ski, or perform an intense battle with an opponent, you will be able to find a game that will let you do just that.

The fighting or boxing games really get the calories burning and keep your heart rate elevated for extended periods of time.

Sporting games, such as those that include skiing, basketball, baseball, or golfing, not only make you sweat, but can also improve your agility, balance, and handeye coordination.

If you are someone who is looking for mind–body benefits or who wants to work on your flexibility, there are a number of yoga games that are also available that are perfect for that.

These games will keep you looking forward to your cardio because they're actually *fun*—and especially when you're playing with a friend! Don't be surprised if time flies and you get in an hour of intense exercise without even realizing it.

Another nice thing about these games is that they reduce the fatigue that you feel because you get so mentally involved in the game that you stop paying attention to the growing exhaustion in your body.

So, hit Amazon and check out your options (I think the best games are on the Nintendo Wii and Microsoft Xbox). Find something that sounds good and give it a try! I think you'll like it!

14

HEAT THINGS UP WITH HOT YOGA

CALORIES BURNED:

300 – 500 per hour

MOST PEOPLE THINK OF YOGA as a form of relaxed stretching, but they probably haven't tried hot yoga before.

Hot yoga is an excellent way to get in cardio training, really work up a sweat and cleanse and detoxify the body, and help build muscle strength while improving your flexibility.

Hot yoga has you do a series of different poses and stretches in a room that's heated to 95–100 degrees (Fahrenheit, of course). A nice thing about exercising in such heat is that it will naturally cause the muscles to loosen and become more limber, which will then allow you to reach new states of flexibility.

Yoga is also a good choice for those who want a trim and lean look, but don't want any muscular bulk. All yoga exercises use your body weight, which can tone your muscles, but won't lead to rapid muscle gain.

When participating in hot yoga, do make sure that you drink plenty of fluids before, during, and especially after the class has finished. This form of exercise is very dehydrating because of all the sweating, so ensure you replace those fluids.

Finally, keep in mind that there are different varieties of hot yoga that you can perform, including Bikram yoga, Vinyasa yoga, Moksha, and power yoga, with each variety offering slightly different benefits. If you're looking for the most intense yoga experience, one that will really jack up your heart rate, hot power yoga is for you.

Hot yoga is a great way to get in cardio and increase flexibility, and I recommend you incorporate it into your training routine!

15

JUMP ROPING

CALORIES BURNED:

400 – 800 per hour

JUMP ROPING IS AN OFTEN-OVERLOOKED form of cardio training that can really work wonders for your body. It's also incredibly convenient because you can do it in the comfort of your own home, and it doesn't require any fancy equipment.

Jump roping not only burns a ton of calories and works your lower body, but it also gets your arms and shoulders working, strengthening them too. You'll also improve your hand–eye coordination and will probably have fun learning different variations of jumps.

You can pick up a rope from your local superstore or fitness store, and it shouldn't cost you any more than $15–20. I recommend that you have a good pair of running shoes, and that you do it on a surface softer than cement, such as carpet, grass, or a wooden floor (this is easier on your knees, ankles, and lower back).

If you're relatively new to working out, shoot for being able to jump rope for five minutes straight. Then take a breather and walk around the room for between three and five minutes, and then go for another five-minute round of jumping. Once you can do this four times, try to do 10 minutes of jumping in your next workout, followed by a rest, and then another 10-minute jumping period.

Once you've got the basic movement down, add in some variety! For example, you could do front jumps for a minute; then back jumps for a minute; then double jumps for a minute; and then one-foot jumps for the final two minutes. Knee-high jumps are also a great variation that will really get your heart pumping.

Have patience while you're learning; jump roping can be a bit tricky at first while you're learning to get coordinated and fast. Spend some time working on your technique before you push yourself hard.

16

THE DRILL SERGEANT ROUTINE

CALORIES BURNED:

650 – 750 per hour

IF YOU'RE LOOKING FOR A WORKOUT program that will challenge muscles that you didn't even realize you had, look no further than this Drill Sergeant Routine.

To perform this workout routine, you'll need to find an open field or large space that is at least a 30-second run from end to end. Ideally, you'd also have a bar of some kind to do pull-ups on (if you want to do this workout at home, you can get a doorway pull-up bar).

So, here's how this routine works: You begin the session by sprinting for about 30 seconds at full speed (run like your life is on the line!). I recommend having a stopwatch so you can time this.

Once you've finished the sprint, you immediately perform 20–40 push-ups (do them until you hit 40 or until you fail). You then perform a dog walk or crab walk (look these up online if you're not sure what they are) back to where you started your sprint. Once you arrive, take a breather for about a minute.

You then sprint again, but this time, do 20–40 sit-ups after instead of the push-ups, followed by a dog or crab walk back and a rest. Do this two more times, with pull-ups and squats as your post-sprint exercises. If you're feeling up for more, start again with push-ups and work your way through the routine a second time.

As you perform these dog and crab walks, make sure that you keep your hips elevated at all times. The biggest mistake that people make when performing these crab or dog walks is allowing the hips to drop, which will then place their lower back at risk of strain.

This is a very intense cardio workout—beginners will probably not be able to finish the whole thing. Do as much as you can, and do a little more next time—and a little more next time—until you can do the whole routine.

17

TRAIN LIKE THE BRITISH ARMY

CALORIES BURNED:

700 – 1200 per hour

YOU'D BE HARD PRESSED TO find groups that know more about physical conditioning than the world's elite armies. When people's lives depend upon their physical and mental endurance and overall fitness, they get pretty serious about working out. In this chapter, we're going to talk about a staple exercise of the British Army—*tabbing*.

"Tabbing" is a contraction of "Tactical Advance to Battle," and it's basically a brisk walk interspersed with periods of running…but with a weighted backpack.

For infantry, the goal is to carry 55 pounds of weight in a backpack for eight miles in less than two hours. I would recommend that you start with a 30-pound pack, and shoot for four miles in an hour. That may not sound like much at first, but the weight combined with the pace required can be quite exhausting.

The pace I recommend to start is to walk briskly for ten minutes, and then run for five minutes; walk for ten minutes, and then run for five, etc.

But as your endurance improves, play a game with yourself: could you make the cut as a British soldier? A 55-pound pack and eight miles in under two hours. To track your distance and time, I recommend using a cardio app on your phone or iPod (there are many great options that keep track of everything for you).

This activity can be especially nice if you have a beautiful countryside to hike through. Because of the slower pace than the typical run, you get to take in the sights a bit more.

Before you hit the asphalt (or better yet, the trails), I want to share a few tips with you. The first is regarding footwear. I recommend boots that support your ankles, and ensure that they are already worn in (new boots will give you painful blisters quickly). Wear thick socks to keep your feet dry, as you'll be sweating quite a bit.

Next is your posture. The weight carried can cause you to hunch forward as you become tired, which will make the activity harder and put strain on your lower back. You should aim to keep your head up, your back straight, and take long strides.

Finally, make sure you use a backpack that has a spine and is built for carrying weight (such as a hiking pack). Also, ensure that the weight in your pack is evenly distributed and isn't heavier on one side than the other.

18

THE CARDIO CORE BLAST

CALORIES BURNED:

400 – 550 per hour

ONE OF THE HALLMARKS OF BEING in shape is having a lean, toned stomach. To accomplish this, you need to have a low percentage of body fat, and also need to develop your ab muscles so they show (to whatever degree you want them to).

A good core-strengthening workout program will be essential for toning or building the midsection, preventing lower back pain, and also warding off injuries that can be caused by a weak core (exercises like squats and deadlifts rely on a strong core for proper form).

This workout focuses on both burning calories and engaging your core, helping you develop strong, chiseled abs that show.

For this workout, you alternate between high-intensity cardio training (which means you go full-out, as hard as you can push yourself) and lower-intensity core training. The core training will serve as a "rest" from the cardio training, and should bring your heart rate down slightly so you can do another cardio interval.

Those who are just starting out and at the beginner level should aim for 30-second cardio intervals and then one minute for the core work. Do this for 20–25 minutes and you'll be wiped.

Those who are better conditioned should aim for one-minute cardio and core intervals for 20–25 total minutes of working out.

Finally, those who are really looking to push themselves should do one-minute cardio intervals and 30-second core workouts. This will be incredibly intense as the cardio training will now dominate the workout, keeping your heart rate elevated the entire time. If you can work up to 20–25 minutes of this, you'll be in *very* good shape.

Because you want to hit your top speed when doing the cardio intervals, sprinting outside works great. But if you can't run for whatever reason, then any other form of cardio will work as long as you push yourself hard. Jump roping is particularly good for this workout.

For the core training, you have several exercises to choose from. I like to move through them, doing a new one each interval. The following exercises are generally recognized as the most effective for strengthening your core:

- Captain's Chair Leg Raise

- Bicycle Crunch

- Crunch

- Cable Crunch

- Ab Wheel

I like this workout because it lets me get in both my abs and cardio at the same time. Give it a try!

BONUS REPORT

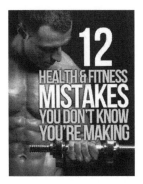

12 HEALTH AND FITNESS MISTAKES YOU DON'T KNOW YOU'RE MAKING

Do you believe that your genetics are preventing you from making great gains in the gym?

Do you do certain exercises because they're supposed to "shape" your muscles?

Do you stretch before lifting weights to prevent injury or increase strength?

When doing cardio, do you shoot for a "target" heart rate zone to burn the most fat possible?

If you answered "yes" to any of those questions, you're in good company as most people do the same.

But here's the kicker: *There's NO science behind any of it.*

Quite to the contrary, however, science actually *disproves* these things.

If you want to learn the truth about these myths and 8 others that ruin people's efforts to get fit, click the link below to download a free bonus report that I put together for you called 12 Health & Fitness Mistakes You Don't Know You're Making.

Visit <u>WWW.BIT.LY/CS-BONUS-REPORT</u> to get this report now!

WOULD YOU DO ME A FAVOR?

Thank you for buying my book. I'm positive that if you just follow what I've written, you will be on your way to looking and feeling better than you ever have before.

I have a small favor to ask. Would you mind taking a minute to write a blurb on Amazon about this book? I check all my reviews and love to get feedback (that's the real pay for my work—knowing that I'm helping people).

Visit the following page to leave me a review:

WWW.AMZN.TO/CS-REVIEW

Also, if you have any friends or family that might enjoy this book, spread the love and lend it to them!

Now, I don't just want to sell you a book—I want to see you use what you've learned to build the body of your dreams.

As you work toward your goals, however, you'll probably have questions or run into some difficulties. I'd like to be able to help you with these, so let's connect up! I don't charge for the help, of course, and I answer questions from readers every day.

Here's how we can connect:

Facebook: facebook.com/muscleforlifefitness

Twitter: @muscleforlife

G+: gplus.to/MuscleForLife

And last but not least, my website is www.muscleforlife.com and if you want to write me, my email address is mike@muscleforlife.com.

Thanks again and I wish you the best!

Mike

P.S. Turn to the next page to check out other books of mine that you might like!

NO PROPRIETARY BLENDS... NO PSEUDOSCIENCE... NO UNDERDOSING KEY INGREDIENTS... REAL WORKOUT SUPPLEMENTS THAT WORK!

HERE'S THE BOTTOM-LINE TRUTH OF THIS MULTI-BILLION-DOLLAR INDUSTRY:

While certain supplements can help, they do NOT build great physiques (proper training and nutrition does), and most are a complete waste of money.

Too many products are "proprietary blends" of low-quality ingredients, junk fillers, and unnecessary additives. Key ingredients are horribly underdosed. There's a distinct lack of credible scientific evidence to back up the outrageous claims made on labels and in ads. The list of what's wrong with this industry goes on and on.

And that's why I decided to get into the supplement game.

What gives? Am I just a hypocritical sell-out? Well, hear me out for a minute and then decide. The last thing we need is yet another marketing machine churning out yet another line of hyped up, flashy products claiming to be more effective than steroids.

I think things should be done differently, and that's why I started LEGION.

Here's what sets LEGION apart from the rabble:

✔ **100% transparent product formulas**

The only reason to use proprietary blends is fraud and deception. You deserve to know exactly what you're buying.

✔ **100% science-based ingredients and dosages**

Every ingredient we use is backed by published scientific literature and is included at true clinically effective dosages.

✔ **100% naturally sweetened with stevia**

Research suggests that regular consumption of artificial sweeteners can be harmful to our health, which is why we use stevia, a natural sweetener with proven health benefits.

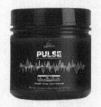
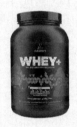
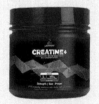
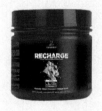

ALSO BY MICHAEL MATTHEWS

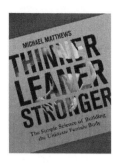

Thinner Leaner Stronger: The Simple Science of Building the Ultimate Female Body

If you want to be toned, lean, and strong as quickly as possible without crash dieting, "good genetics," or wasting ridiculous amounts of time in the gym and money on supplements...*regardless of your age...* then you want to read this book.

Visit www.muscleforlife.com to get this book!

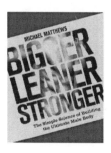

Bigger Leaner Stronger: The Simple Science of Building the Ultimate Male Body

If you want to be muscular, lean, and strong as quickly as possible, without steroids, "good genetics," or wasting ridiculous amounts of time in the gym, and money on supplements...then you want to read this book.

Visit www.muscleforlife.com to get this book!

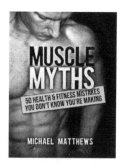

Muscle Myths: 50 Health & Fitness Mistakes You Don't Know You're Making

If you've ever felt lost in the sea of contradictory training and diet advice out there and you just want to know once and for all what works and what doesn't—what's scientifically true and what's false—when it comes to building muscle and getting ripped, then you need to read this book.

Visit www.muscleforlife.com to get this book!

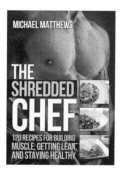

The Shredded Chef: 120 Recipes for Building Muscle, Getting Lean, and Staying Healthy

If you want to know how to forever escape the dreadful experience of "dieting" and learn how to cook nutritious, delicious meals that make building muscle and burning fat easy and enjoyable, then you need to read this book.

Visit www.muscleforlife.com to get this book!

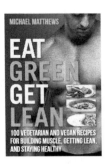

Eat Green Get Lean: 100 Vegetarian and Vegan Recipes for Building Muscle, Getting Lean, and Staying Healthy

If you want to know how to build muscle and burn fat by eating delicious vegetarian and vegan meals that are easy to cook and easy on your wallet, then you want to read this book.

Visit www.muscleforlife.com to learn more about this book!

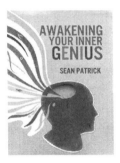

Awakening Your Inner Genius

If you'd like to know what some of history's greatest thinkers and achievers can teach you about awakening your inner genius, and how to find, follow, and fulfill your journey to greatness, then you want to read this book today.

(I'm using a pen name for this book, as well as for a few other projects not related to health and fitness, but I thought you might enjoy it so I'm including it here.)

Visit www.yourinnergenius.com to learn more about this book!

Made in the USA
San Bernardino, CA
22 May 2014